CAMBRIDGE LIBRARY COLLECTION

Books of enduring scholarly value

History of Medicine

It is sobering to realise that as recently as the year in which On the Origin of Species was published, learned opinion was that diseases such as typhus and cholera were spread by a 'miasma', and suggestions that doctors should wash their hands before examining patients were greeted with mockery by the profession. The Cambridge Library Collection reissues milestone publications in the history of Western medicine as well as studies of other medical traditions. Its coverage ranges from Galen on anatomical procedures to Florence Nightingale's common-sense advice to nurses, and includes early research into genetics and mental health, colonial reports on tropical diseases, documents on public health and military medicine, and publications on spa culture and medicinal plants.

An Historiall Expostulation against the Beastlye Abusers, Both of Chyrurgerie and Physyke, in Oure Tyme

The surgeon Thomas Pettigrew (1791–1865) was interested in all aspects of antiquity. He gained fame in society through his mummy-unwrapping parties, and his *History of Egyptian Mummies* is also reissued in the Cambridge Library Collection. His interest in the early history of medicine is evidenced by this edition of a work by John Hall, which was published by the Percy Society in 1844. Hall was a surgeon, born 1529/30, who published this work in 1565 as an appendix to his translation of the work of the thirteenth-century surgeon Lanfranc of Milan. Little is known about Hall except that he practised medicine in Maidstone, Kent, and had published acrostic verses. He was vociferous in his indignation against fraudulent medicine, and this work describes nine incidents where quacks, both male and female, had visited Maidstone and offered miraculous cures to the gullible: Hall himself was involved in prosecuting some of them.

Cambridge University Press has long been a pioneer in the reissuing of out-of-print titles from its own backlist, producing digital reprints of books that are still sought after by scholars and students but could not be reprinted economically using traditional technology. The Cambridge Library Collection extends this activity to a wider range of books which are still of importance to researchers and professionals, either for the source material they contain, or as landmarks in the history of their academic discipline.

Drawing from the world-renowned collections in the Cambridge University Library and other partner libraries, and guided by the advice of experts in each subject area, Cambridge University Press is using state-of-the-art scanning machines in its own Printing House to capture the content of each book selected for inclusion. The files are processed to give a consistently clear, crisp image, and the books finished to the high quality standard for which the Press is recognised around the world. The latest print-on-demand technology ensures that the books will remain available indefinitely, and that orders for single or multiple copies can quickly be supplied.

The Cambridge Library Collection brings back to life books of enduring scholarly value (including out-of-copyright works originally issued by other publishers) across a wide range of disciplines in the humanities and social sciences and in science and technology.

An Historiall Expostulation

against the Beastlye Abusers,
Both of Chyrurgerie
and Physyke, in Oure Tyme

With a Goodlye Doctrine and Instruction,
Necessarye to be Marked and Followed,
of All True Chirurgiens

JOHN HALL
EDITED BY T.J. PETTIGREW

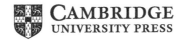

CAMBRIDGE
UNIVERSITY PRESS

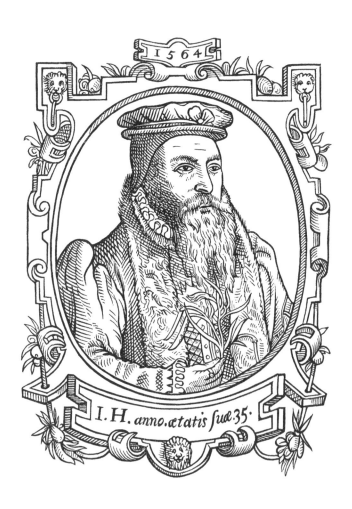

I. H. anno. ætatis ſuæ 35.

AN

Historiall Expostulation:

AGAINST

THE BEASTLYE ABUSERS, BOTH OF CHYRURGERIE

AND PHYSYKE, IN OURE TYME:

WITH

A goodlye Doctrine and Instruction,

NECESSARYE TO BE MARKED AND FOLOWED,

OF ALL TRUE CHIRURGIENS:

BY

JOHN HALLE,

CHYRURGYEN.

———

EDITED BY

T. J. PETTIGREW, ESQ., F.R.S., F.S.A.

FELLOW OF THE ROYAL COLLEGE OF SURGEONS OF ENGLAND,
DOCTOR OF PHILOSOPHY OF THE UNIVERSITY OF GÜTTINGEN,
ETC. ETC. ETC.

———

LONDON.

PRINTED FOR THE PERCY SOCIETY,

BY T. RICHARDS, 100, ST. MARTIN'S LANE.

———

M.DCCC.XLIV.

INTRODUCTION.

THE following tract is appended to a rare work which forms one of the earliest English books in surgery. It is a translation of Lanfranc's "Chirurgia Parva," by John Hall, surgeon. Of the translator little is known. There are no biographical notices of him beyond those which can be gathered from his writings, and from these we learn that he was a surgeon in practice at Maidstone, in Kent, and a "member of the worshipful Company of Chirurgeons." He addresses his book to the members of that body, for protection, as well as to call upon them to unite with him in his endeavours to put down empiricism, and to advance the knowledge of surgeons in general. He appears to have been a man of strong mind, and of great zeal in his profession. A portrait, (wood cut), of which a facsimile is here given, taken when thirty-five years of age, shows that he was born in 1529 or 1530, and is prefixed to the work.

Following his " Vera Effigies," is, in seven quatrains :—

THE BOOKES VERDICT.

As some delighte moste to beholde,
  Eche newe devyse and guyse,
So some in workes of fathers olde,
  Their studies exercise.

Perusing with all diligence
  Bokes written long before :
Wherin they learne experience,
  To heale both sicke and sore ;

Which I alowe in dede and werde,
  In those that understande ;
For otherwyse it is a sworde
  Put in a mad mans hande.

Let idiotes and betles blynde,
  Therefore lay me aparte :
Leste contrarie myne author's mynde
  They rudly me perverte.

For as the bee doth honie take
  From every goodly flowre,
And spyders of the same doe make
  Venim that wyll devoure :

So all that learned men and wyse
  To good purpose can use,
The rude, that knowledge doe despise,
  Will ever more abuse.

Wherefore all those that use me right
  I shall increase their fame :
And vyle abusers all my mighte
  Shall be to doe them shame.

In his address "unto the Worshipful the Maisters, Wardens, and consequently to all the whole
Company and Brotherhood of Chirurgiens of London," he strongly laments the prevalent ignorance
of the profession, "and alas," says he, "where as
there is one in Englande, almoste throughout al
the realme, that is indede a true minister of this
arte, there are tenne abhominable abusers of the
same. Where as there is one chirurgien that was
apprentise to his arte, or one physicien that hath
travayled in the true studie and exercise of phisique,
there are tenne that are presumptious swearers,
smatterers, or abusers of the same ; yea, smythes,
cutlers, carters, coblars, copers, coriars of lether,
carpenters, and a great rable of women." He
afterwards says, " I would to God, therfore, my
dere maisters and brethren, that there might no
fault be found in us concerning these thinges ; for
truly if we weare such men of science as we ought
to be, these false abusers would be more fearful to
medle as they doe." He contrasts the conduct
and information of the professors of other arts and
sciences, with those of surgery, and he demon-
strates the necessity of drawing attention to the
works of the learned and experienced, to improve
their condition. With this view he undertook the
translation of Lanfranc's work.

LANFRANC was a physician, born at Milan, and

flourished in the thirteenth century. He was a
pupil of Gulielmus de Saliceto, and having com-
pleted his studies, he went into France and settled
at Lyons, whence he was, by his great reputation,
called to Paris, where he taught his profession
with great *éclat*. His work is intitled " Ars Chi-
rurgica," the MS. of which is in the Bibliothèque
du Roi de France. It gives a miserable picture of
the state of surgery in France in his time, and
was first published at Venice, in 1490, and again
in 1519, and 1546. It was also printed at Lyons,
in 1553, together with the works of Guy de Chauliac, Roger, &c., and it was translated into Ger-
man by Otho Brunfels, and published at Frankfort
in 1566. Altogether it is of little importance,
and relates to the " treating of woundes, of apos-
themes, of ulcers, (the cancer and the fistula), of
algebra or restoration, (dislocations and fractures),
and of the diseases of the eyes." Then ensues
" The Antidotarie," or account of remedies em-
ployed, which concludes " Lanfranc's Briefe."
Halle says that it was translated " out of Frenshe,
into the olde Saxony English, about two hundred
years past."

John Halle is bold in his expressions against
the quacks of his day, a most determined enemy
to ignorant empirics, exulting in the exposure of
their nefarious practices, their urinoscopical

examinations, &c., and loud in his protestations against the combination of magic, divination, and physic. In one place he says, "I will not cease while breath is in my body, to lay on with both handes till this battell be wonne, and our adversaries convinced and vanquished; which, although, as I saide afore, they are tenne to one, yet truthe being our weapon, and good science our armoure, with our generall the high author of them, we nede not to doubt but that one shal be good enough for a thousand, not so strongly armed, but naked men, and bare of all knowledge." He seems, however, to have had some misgivings as to the publication of the "Historiall Expostulation," as a letter from Dr. William Cuningham, a reader of lectures at Surgeons' Hall, and dated from his house in Colman Street, April 18th, 1565, is affixed in recommendation of the undertaking, and advises him not to withhold his condemnation of the "rabble of ronnagates." This is succeeded by another letter, from the pen of Thomas Gale, a "maister in chirurgerye," approving his work, and urging its publication in the following manner: " Aspire, therfore, and take breth unto you; let no vayne and frivolous opinion overcome you, for I see no cause wherfore you shoulde excruciate your selfe. Every wyse man wyll accepte your indevours, excepte those whiche neyther mynde theyr office,

neither the utilitie of the publique wealth ; every
good man will embrase, and with great gladnes
revolve over your boke as sone as it is published,
and wil, at the first sight of your good travell,
have you in more estimacion then ever they had.
And why? because you set forth the most famous
and excellent arte of medicine."

Some lines addressed to the "loving readers,"
precede John Halle's own epistle to the reader, in
which occur many good observations, and in
which the character of the man is well displayed.
He lays on most lustily against the empirics, and
ignorant surgions, the "very caterpyliers to the
publique orders." He accuses them of running
about the country, "like pedlars, tynkers, ratte
katchers, and very vacaboundes, some only to set
bones, some to drawe tethe, some to let blood,
some to cutte ruptures, and take out stones ; but
all thys rather (under suche colour), to mayntayne
an idle and thevyshe lyfe, then to profyte the common weale, to the great uprobrie of all the whole
profession of medicine." He then laments that
less attention is paid to the making of good surgeons, than of other artificers. "Alas, there are
goodly orders taken, and profitable lawes made,
for makyng of clothe, tannyng of leather, makyng
of shoes, and many other externall thynges, the
abuse wherof is but a dearth or disprofite of

the purse ; and shall there not be a redresse had
for the true use of a science whereupon dependeth
the health of mans body ? without whiche what is
mans lyfe but a very misery or wretched werines ?
the abuse of whiche science is not only a disprofite
to the purse, but a farre greater charge, that is to
saye, the losse of helth and lyfe." He descants
upon the neglect shown to apprentises taken by
many, as he says, " not for to teache them science,
but only to be their drudge, and to doe their toyle
and labore, which is the cause, that so many come
out of their yeares so ignorant. For their intent
is to have servantes to dooe the toyle in their
house, and not to make them cunnyng men ; yea,
and some will refuse a yonge man that is learned,
and apte to understande, to have an ignorant slave,
to beare the water tankard, and scoure pannes ;
suche a one, (as the common proverbe is), that
will never doe man of science harme, unles he steale
away his dynner."

The necessary consequence of this conduct is
thus pointed out ; " And yet will suche a one
bragge and boaste, at seven years ende, as though
he had all the learnyng and cunnyng under the
sunne, although in very dede, the moste knowledge that he hath is, to poule, or shave, drawe a
toothe, or dresse a broken pate. Alas, is not this
a great pytye, that suche a noble arte shall thus

be abused every way, through the filthie lucre and
avaricious myndes of men? Is it not a shame to
use such roberie? Doe ye not steale lyke robers
the service of your apprentyses, when contrary to
your covenants, ye hyde your science from your
servantes, to whom ye are bounde to teache it;
and yet, (in the meane season), receive the labor
of their bodyes more lyke slaves then men; beside the great dishonor that therby you doe to
your own profession, God graunt that I may see
this amended, as I trust I shall."

Halle objects to the division of medical science,
shows the dependence of the several departments
upon each other, by reference to the opinions of
ancient authors; asserts that by "pernicious
division all hath been brought to confusion, so
that neither parte is nowe used only of the experte
professors therof, but rather of every smearer,
that listeth to abuse them. For as the phy-
siciens thynke their learnyng sufficient, without
practyse or experience, so the chirurgien, for the
moste parte, havyng experience and practise,
thinketh it unnedeful to have any learnyng at all,
which also hath boldened every ignorant rusticall,
ye and foolyshe women, to think them selves
sufficient to profess and worke in so noble and
worthy an arte." He then states what a surgeon
should be: learned, expert, of good discretion, &c.

and having established these points, he asks,
" Why is every rude, rusticke, braynsicke beast,
fond foole, undiscrete idiote; yea every bedlem
baude, and scoldinge drabbe, suffered thus (without all order) to abuse this worthy arte upon the
body of man? What avayleth the goodly orders,
taken by our forefathers and ancient authores,
that none should be admitted to the arte of
chirurgery, that are miscreate or deformed of
body; as goggle or skwynte eyed, unperfecte of
sight, unhelthy of body, unperfecte of mynde, not
hole in his members, boystrous fingers or shakyng
handes. But contrary-wyse, that all that should
be admytted to that arte, should be of cleare and
perfect sight, well formed in person, hole of mynde
and of members, sclender and tender fingered,
havyng a softe and stedfast hande: or as the
common sentence is, a chirurgien should have
three dyvers properties in his person. That is to
saie, a harte as the harte of a lyon, his eyes like
the eyes of an hawke, and his handes as the
handes of a woman: what avayleth this order I
saye, sithe the contrary in all poyntes is put dayly
in use, and that almost without hope of redresse?
seyng also, that those auncient authors had not
only this regarde to the forme of the body, but
also, and as well to the bewtie or ornament of the
mynde, and honest conversation of him that should

be admitted to chirurgery, as are thes : He ought
to be well manered, of good audacitie, and bolde
where he may worke surely ; and, contrariwise,
doubtfull, and fearfull, in things that be dangerous
and desperate. He must be gentyll to his pacients,
witty in prognostications, and forseyng of dangers,
apte and reasonable to answere and dissolve all
doubtes and questions belongynge to his worke.
He muste also be chaste, sober, meeke, and mercifull; no extorcioner, but so to accomplishe his
rewarde, at the handes of the ryche, to maynteine
his science and necessary lyvynges, that he may
helpe the poore for the only sake of God : what
meaneth it, I saye, (those things considered) that
so many sheepe heades, unwytty, unlearned,
unchaste, ribaudes, lecheours, fornicators; dronk-
ardes, belygoddes, beastly gluttons, wrathfull,
envious and evell manered, shall thus myserably
be suffred to abuse so noble an arte ; yea, that
they shall also be mayntayned (in despyght of
those that are men of science indede) proferred
lyvynges for that profession, contrary to the
ordinances and lawes of a citie, beyng a carpenter,
a cobler, or a corier of lether, or whatsoever he be:
the wyttye, the learned, the man of knowledge,
the citizen, and the free man, in the meane season
wantyng preferrement and lyvyng?"

He professes much anxiety for the success of

his observations, and trusts that if his book, being
read by any abuser of chirurgery, he should find
himself "rubbed on the galle," he will leave his
vice and improve. He also admonishes the young
to study, to attend to their anatomy, to the nature
and complexions of their patients, and the properties of their medicines; to let their practise be
founded on their reason, and that "none may
worke without knowledge joyned to experience."
Finally, he warns the young man entering the
profession, to avoid "games and spendyng the
time in playe. And hereof assure thy selfe, that
if thou have not as great desyre to thy boke, as
the greatest gamner hath to his game, thou shalte
never worthily be called cunnyng in this arte.
For thou must thynke and esteme all tyme of
leysure from thy worke and busynes, even loste
and evill bestowed, in which thou hast not pro-
fyted somewhat at thy boke. Let thy boke therefore, I say, be thy pastyme and game: which (if
thou love it as thou oughtest) will so delight thee,
that thou shalt thinke no tyme so well bestowed
as at it. Yea, thou must desyre it as the child
doeth his mother's pappe; and so will it nourishe
thee, that thou shalt worthily growe and increase
to a worshypfull fame of cunnynge and learnyng."
To the work of Lanfranc, Halle has added an
expositive table of the "strange wordes, names,

diseases, symples, &c. which occur in the book;
' A very frutefull and necessary briefe worke of
Anatomie," and the " Historiall Expostulation,"
herewith reprinted. To the first of these is
affixed the following acrostic :—

NOMEN AUTHORIS SUB HIS ATRACTILIS JACET.

If reason maye the justice be
Of this my minde the truthe to trye :
Howe can ther be dispaire in me
No truthe sithe reason can denye.

Happye it is when men esteme :
All one in truthe, the same to tell :
Let no man voyde of reason deme,
Lest he agaynste the truthe rebell.

The proheme contains a very creditable defence
of the ancients and their modes of study, and
concludes with some quaint lines which terminate
thus :—

In wicked men, so wickednes
Will alway have alway :
Dispraising still, throughe hatefulnesse,
Eche good and perfect way.

Thomas Halle, the brother of the author, then
addresses the " Gentle Readers that thirst for
science," and adds several stanzas in praise of the
intent of the work, and also some lines which bear

the signature of "Ihon Yates, Chirurgion." In
the table, under the head of Algebra, is said:
"This Araby worde *Algebra* sygnifyeth as well
fractures, as of bones, &c. as somtyme the
restauratyon of the same." Of Scabiosa "Men
saye that S. Urban at the peticions of a certaine
asthmatike sister of his, (that used scabiosa
continually) sente to hir these verses, of the
vertues therof :—

URBANUS SUO SENESCIT PRETIUM SCABIOSÆ.

Non purgat pectus quod comprimit ægra senectus ;
Lenit pulmonem, purgat laterum regionem ;
Apostema frangit, si locum bibita tangit :
Tribus uncta foris anthracem liberat horis.

To Urbane him selfe, it is uncertaine
Howe many vertues in scabiose reygne :
But excellently it clenseth the breste
Of sicke aged folke, that there are opreste.

The pypes of the lunges, if rough they apere,
It maketh them smothe, yea gentle and clere ;
The roumes of the breste, that we the sydes call,
It purgeth well, from incumbrances all.

If it be drunke, so that it touche the place,
Apostemes it breakes, by peculiar grace ;
Without to carbuncles if it layde be,
It doth lose and breake them within howres three."

XX

At the end of the table are these verses :—

> Though envie me accuse,
>   In suche as wyll disdayne;
> It can not make me muse,
>   Nor nothyng rere my brayne.
>
> For they that doe misuse
>   Their tongues in suche a case,
> Wyll styll them selves abuse,
>   In runnyng of that rase.
>
> But reason is myne ayde
>   To take my cause in hande:
> And I nothyng afrayde
>   With hir in place to stande.
>
> Havyng my hope so stayde,
>   That those who lyste to rayle
> Wyllbe ryght sore dismayde,
>   When reason shall prevayle.
>
> For truthe, by reason strong,
>   Wyll have the upper hande;
> When envie vyle and wronge,
>   Shall fayntly flee the lande.
>
> And truthe hath alwaye been,
>   A daughter unto tyme;
> Whiche as it hath been seen,
>   Detecteth every cryme.

The " Treatise of Anatomie" forms the principal work of our author. He quotes from a writer, Henricus de Ermunda Villa, who compareth

" the chirurgien ignorant in anatomy, to a blynde
man whiche woude hewe a pece of tymber; for
as a blynd man that heweth on a logge knoweth
not how muche he should hewe therof, nor in what
maner, (and therfore commonly erreth in hewyng
more or lesse than he ought to doe :) so lyke wyse
doth the chyrurgien that worketh on the body of
man, not knowing the anatomy." The frame of
man, he tells us, has been called by the Greeks
" Microcosmos, a little world, because in the same
(even as in the frame of the greate worlde) so
manye wonders maye bee seene of natures works
to the hygh honor and glorye of Almyghtye God.
Maye it not be proved, that the brayne (lyke unto
the heavens) hangeth without any maner of staye
or proppe, to holde by the same ? nay, it is so
evident, that every learned anatomiste writeth
of the same, as a thyng not to be doubted of, and
therfore judge the same to have a certeyne lyke-
nes with the heavenly nature. And as the world
hath two notable lyghtes to governe the same,
namely, the sonne and the moone; so hath the
body of man, planted lykewyse in the hyghest
place, twoo lyghtes, called eyes, whiche are the
lyghtes of the body, as the sonne and the moone
are the lyghtes of the world. And it is also
wrytten of some doctors, that the brayne hath vii
concavites, being instrumentes of the wyttes,

which answere unto the vii spheres of the planetes.
And to be briefe, it is a worlde to beholde, and a
wonderful wonder to thynke, that as great mer-
veyles may bee seene, wrought by God in nature
in this little worlde, man his body, as ther is to
be considered in any thyng in the unyversall great
worlde, above or benethe at any tyme.

" Secondly, it is called a common weale, for as
muche as there is therin conteyned as it were a
ryghteous regiment, betwene a prynce and his
subjectes, as for example.   Let us call the harte
of man a king, the brayne and the lyver the chiefe
governours under hym, the stomache and the
guttes, with other aperteinyng to nutryments, the
officers of his courte, and all the members
universally his subjectes.   And then let us see, if
any man can devyse any necessary instrument of
a common weale, nedefull for the wealth of the
same, from the hyghest to the lowest, that the
lyke shall not be founde in the body of man, as
it is so well knowne to all those that travel in the
knowledge of anatomie, that I nede not here
muche therof to wryte.   Can it be perceyved that
the hande or the fote, or any part of them or such
lyke (which we may lyken to the labourers, or as
some call them vyle members of a common weale)
at any tyme to resiste or rebel againste the harte
their soveraigne lord, or any other officer under

hym their superiors? No, truly. The body of
man is a common weale without rebellion: the
kyng so lovyng his subjectes, and the subjectes so
lovyng their kyng, that the one is ever redy to
mynister unto the other all thynges nedeful; as
if the harte by any occasion susteyne damage, as
we may see in the disease called *Sincope,* or
swoundyng. At suche a tyme I saye the face, the
handes, and the fete, are founde colde and without
felynge, strengthe or lyfe; and what proveth it,
but that as lovynge and obedient subjectes they
thynke nothyng theyr own wherof the harte hath
nede, which is their lorde and governour; yea,
they utterly depryve themselves of altogether to
serve and please their lord. Immediately as the
swoundyng ceaseth, the bloude resorteth to the
face, the handes and the feete are warme agayne,
as it were benefittes done, rendered agayne with
thankes and joye. And is not such a lorde and
kyng worthye of good subjectes, that for the helpe
of one of the leaste of them wyl spend all that he
hath, so long as lyfe endureth? as if a member be
hurte, wherby any veyne or artery is cutte, the
bloude or spirit will issue in suche wyse that it
wyll not cease commyng thyther so longe as any
is lefte, if it be not in tyme prevented. Oh kynd
and gentyll governour, oh wel wyllyng and obedient subjectes."

His anatomy is composed to the end of advancing his chirurgery, and for the time in which it was written, is a very fair compendium. There are two figures whole length, cut in wood, but the references apply only to the exterior parts of the body and its regions. The conclusion of the work gives a good summary in relation to the temperaments. All his writings appear to be terminated by rhyming verses, and those attached to his anatomy are in praise of chirurgery, as founded upon a knowledge of anatomy, and condemnation of those who practise without learning.

Halle's antipathy to quacks was inveterate. Throughout his writings he omits no opportunity of expressing his horror of, and aversion to them ; but in the following and concluding " Historiall Expostulation," he enters into particulars, gives many curious details of the practices of itinerant impostors, principally such as resided in, or visited Maidstone, in Kent, where it appears he exercised his profession. His " Goodlye Doctrine and Instruction" is drawn up in verse, and is marked by good sense, and in itself is a curious composition.

According to Watt and other authorities, Hall or Halle was also author of " The Court of Virtue, containing many Holy or Spretual Songs, Sonnettes, Psalmes, Ballets, and Shorte Sentences, as well as of Holy Scripture as others, with Music, Notes, London, 1565," 16mo.

But an earlier production, (being in 1550), may be mentioned : " Certayne Chapters taken out of the Proverbes of Solomon, with other Chapters of the Holy Scripture, and certayne Psalmes of David, translated into English Metre, by John Hall." By the remainder of the title it appears that the proverbs had been, in a former impression, unfairly attributed to Thomas Sternhold.

A copy of verses by Halle, is prefixed to " The Enchiridion of Surgery, by Thomas Gale, London, 1563, 12mo." Halle and Gale seem to have enjoyed much intimacy, and to have had minds congenial to each other. Gale served in the army of Henry VIII, at Montreal, in 1544, and in that of King Philip, at St. Quintin, in 1557 ; he was serjeant-surgeon to Queen Elizabeth, and his picture of the state of military surgery in his time, appears to have been no better than the civil surgery as described by Halle. The following extract may not be uninteresting to the reader :—

" I remember," says he, "when I was in the wars," in the time of that most famous prince, King Henry VIII, there was a great rabblement there, that took upon them to be surgeons. Some were sow-gelders, and some horse-gelders, with tinkers and coblers. This noble sect did such great cures that they got themselves a perpetual name ; for, like as Thessalus's sect were called Thessalians, so

d

was this rabblement, for their notorious cures,
called dog-leachers, for in two dressings they did
commonly make their cures whole and sound for
ever, so that they neither felt heat nor cold, nor
no manner of pain after. But when the Duke of
Norfolk, who was then general, understood how
the people did die, and that of small wounds, he
sent for me and certain other surgeons, command-
ing us to make search how these men came to
their death, whether it were by the grevousness of
their wounds, or by the lack of knowledge of the
surgeons ; and we, according to our command-
ment, made search through all the camp, and
found many of the same good fellows, which took
upon them the names of surgeons,—not only the
names but the wages also. We asking of them
whether they were surgeons, or no, they said they
were ; we demanded with whom they were brought
up, and they with shameless faces would answer,
either with one cunning man or another, who was
dead. Then we demanded of them what chirurgery stuff they had to cure men withal, and
they would show us a pot or a box, which they had
in a budget, wherein was such trumpery as they
did use to grease horses heels withal, and laid
upon scabbed horses backs, with nerval, and such
like. And other that were coblers and tinkers,
they used shoe maker's wax, with the rust of old

pans, and made therewithal a noble salve, as they did term it. But in the end this worthy rabble-ment was committed to the Marshalsea, and threatened by the duke's grace to be hanged for their worthy deeds, except they would declare the truth what they were, and of what occupations, and in the end they did confess, as I have declared to you before."

The Bodleian Library contains a MS. (178), being a translation by J. H. of Bened. Victorius's " Cure of the French Disease"; also some letters between J. H. and Dr. William Cuningham, dated 1565. The latter is well known by his " Cosmographical Glasse, containing the pleasant principles of Cosmographie, Geographie, Hydrographie, or Navigation, London, 1559, folio." Many of the cuts of this work were executed by the author, who is reported to have been ingenious in the art of engraving on copper; the map of ' Norwich' is his own production. The work is one of the finest that issued from the press of Day. Mr. Halliwell tells me that a few years ago he saw the original MS. of this work at Denley's, a bookseller, near Drury Lane. Dr. Cuningham resided at Norwich about 1556-59, and afterwards in London, where he was appointed to read the lectures at Surgeon's Hall, in 1563. He commented on the book of Galen upon " Tumours against Nature."

xxviii

He also wrote a Commentary on the book " De
Aere Aquis et Regionibus," by Hippocrates.   He
calls Morbus Gallicus *Chamæleontiasis.*

T. J. P.

AN

HISTORIALL EXPOSTULATION:

Against the beastlye Abusers, bothe of Chyrurgerie,
and Physyke, in oure tyme: with a goodlye
Doctrine and Instruction, necessarye to
be marked and folowed, of all true
Chirurgiens:

Gathered and diligently set forth

by

JOHN HALLE, Chyrurgyen.

Imprinted at London in Flete Streate, nyghe unto Saint Dun-
stones Churche, by Thomas Marshe.

An. 1565.

AN

HYSTORIALL EXPOSTULATION,

ETC.

For as muche as in the epistle and prefaces, I have declared the dishonor that the noble arte of medicyne susteyneth by deceavynge fugitives, and other false abusers ; I thinke it good here to blasen the dedes of some in this our tyme, that it maye apere that not withoute a sufficiente cause, I have so there of them complayned.

Fyrst, there came into the towne of Maydstone, in the yere of our Lorde, 1555, a woman whiche named hir selfe Jone, havyng with hir a walkyng mate whome she called her husbande. This wicked beast toke hir inne at the sygne of the Bell, in the towne aforesayde, where she caused within short space to be published that she could heale all maner, bothe inward and out-ward diseases. One powder she caried in a blader, made of the herbe daphnoydes, and anise sede together, whiche shee (as an onelye sufficient remedie for all grefes), administred unto all hir folishe patientes, in lyke quantite to all people, neyther regardyng tyme,

B 2

strengthe, nor age. All the tyme of her being there, (whiche was about iii wekes), there resorted to her company, divers ruffians, and vacaboundes, under pretence of being diseased, and sekyng to her for remedye, so that hir false profession, was unto their wicked behavioure, for the tyme in that towne a safe supportation.

This beastlie deceaver, amonge manie others, tooke in hand an honest mans child, who had a suppurat tumor in his navell, percynge dangerouslye the panicles of the belye, to whome she administered the sayde pouder in great quantitye, in so muche, that the childe dyd vomyte continuallye for the space of halfe a daye and more, withoute ceassynge, whereby the sayde aposteme brake.

The parentes of the chylde then feared much, by the grevousnesse of the syghte, that his stomache woulde breake, whiche may be thought that in very dede it so dyd. For in processe of tyme ther issued out by the orifice of the same vii. wormes, at vii. severall tymes (such as children are wont to avoyde eyther upwarde or downwarde, from the stomache and guttes, called *teretes i. rotundi*), with also a certayne yelowe substance, not stinkynge, suche as we sometymes fynde in the stomaches of dead men when we open them.

This fearfull syght, I saye, caused the childes parentes to sende for me, to knowe therein myne opinion and counsell; unto whome I prognosticated (as I sawe good cause), that the mater was very dangerous, and not lyke to be cured. But this beastly forme of a woman, hearyng me so saye, answered that she douted therein no daunger, and farthermore offered hirselfe to be locked up in a chamber with the chylde, and that yf she healed him not, shee myghte be punished; with a great deale more circumstance of prating and deceyt-full braggynge werdes.   Unto whose moste wicked and divlishe boldnes I thus answered.   Wher as you saye that ye doubte not any daunger in this childe, I verye well beleue you, for ignorante fooles can doubte no perils, and who is bolder then blynde bayerd? howe shoulde they doubte that knowe not what a doubt meaneth?   Notwithstandyng this preheminence you deceavynge rennegates have, ye maye bragge, lye, and face, tyll ye have murdered, or destroyed suche as cre-dyte you, and then are ye gone, ye shewe your heles, and that is onelye your defence.   But honest menne of arte muste have truthe for theyr defence, and expe-rience of their true worke, and maye promyse no more then they may performe.

What should I make manye wordes, the parentes of the childe all to late discharged this deceaver, and the child, notwithstandyng the counsell had of dyvers learned men, dyed afterwarde of the sayde grefe.   But the sayde deceaver, accordyng to my prophesie, after iii. dayes, ran away, she and her walkyng mate, rob-bynge their hoste where they lay, of the shetes, pillow-beres, and blankets that they laye in; and by their entysement of one of the mayde servauntes of their sayd hoste, they hadde muscadell served them insteade of bere, whyle they laye there for the moste parte;

which entyced servant ranne awaye also with them, and coulde not synce be herde of.

Secondly, in the yere of our Lord 1556, there resorted unto Maydstone, one Robert Haris, professynge and pretendyng an hyghe knowlege in physike; under cloke wherof he deceaved mervaylouslie with vyle sorcerie. This deceaver could tel (as the folish people reported of hym), by only lokyng in ones face, all secrete markes and scarres of the bodie, and what they had done, and what hadde chaunced unto them all theyr lyfe tyme before. Wherwith he had so incensed the fonde and waveryng myndes of some, that pitie was to here. Amonge whome one woman (whoe for hir yeares and profession, ought to have bene more discrete). When I reasoned with hir agaynste his doynges, she ernestlie affirmed that she knewe well that he was then dystant from hir, at the leaste vii. myles, and yet she verelye beleved that he knewe what she then sayde. Oh greate beastlynes and infydelitie, specially in suche as have borne a face to favour the worde of God.

Well, for jestyng a lyttell agaynste the madnes of thys deceaver, I hadde a dagger drawne at me not longe after. The wordes that I spake were to his hostes, when I sawe him goe by, in this wyse. Is this (quod I), the cunnyng sothsayer, that is sayde to lye at your house? Sothesayer, quod shee; I knowe no suche thynge by him, therefore ye are to blame so to name him. Why, quod I, suche men and suche enformed me that he can tell of thynges loste, and helpe children and cattell bewitched and forspoken, and can tell by lokyng in ones face, what markes he hathe on his bodie, and where, and tell them what they have done, and their fortune to come.   Yea, and all this in dede he can doe, quod she.   Why, then, he is a sothe-sayer and a sorcerer, quod I.   Well, quod she, yf he have so muche cunnynge in his bellye, he is the hap-pyer, and it is the more joye of him.   Nay, quod I, it were mere folyshnes for hym to carye his cunnyng in his bellye.   And why? quod she.   Why, quod I, thynke you that men of lerning and knowledge cary their cunnynge in their bellies?   Wher else, quod she, and why not?   Mary, quod I, yf he should beare his cunnyng there, he should alwayes waste it when he wente to the privye, and so in time he should lose all his cunnyng.   This beyng merylye spoken, turned me afterwards not to a little displeasure, even at their handes, where I had deserved and loked for frendship as of dutie; but I must cease to marveyle any longer at this, when almoste everie suche abhominable vylaine is de-fended, upholden, and mayntayned, by suche as of righte, and according to the holesome lawes of this realme, shoulde punish them for these their abusions. Yet surelie the grieffe were the lesse, yf onely the blynde, and supersticious antiquitie had a regarde and love to suche deceavers.   But nowe a great number that have borne an outwarde shewe of great holynes, and love to Gods holie worde ; we see them seke day-lie to suche divelishe wyches and sorcerers, if their fynger doe but ake, as though they were Goddes, and coulde presentlie helpe them with wordes, although they knowe that God in his Israell, hath called them an abhominacion, and hath farther commaunded that none suche should be suffred among them to lyve.

Thyrdlie, in the year of our Lord a thousand fyve hundred fyftie and eyght, there came to Maydstone one Thomas Lufkyn, by occupacion a fuller, and burler of clothe, and had bene brought up (by reporte of divers honest men), at the fullyng mylles there besyde the towne, nevertheles he had ben longe absent from that contrie, in whiche tyme he had by roving abroade, become a phisician, a chirurgien, an astronomier, a palmister, a phisiognomier, a sothsayer, a fortune devyner, and I can not tell what. This deceaver was the beastliest beguiler by his sorcerys that euer I herd of, making physike the onely colour to cover all his crafty thefte and mischieves, for he set uppe a byll at hys fyrste commynge, to publishe his beyng there, the tenour wherof was in effect as followeth :—

If anye manne, womanne, or childe bee sicke, or would be let bloud, or bee diseased with anye maner of inward or outwarde grefes, as al maner of agues, or fevers, plurises, cholyke, stone, strangulion, impostumes, fistulas, kanker, goutes, pocks, bone ache, and payne of the joynts, which commeth for lacke of bloudlettyng, let them resorte to the sygne of the Sarazens Hedde, in the easte lane, and brynge theire waters with them to be sene, and they shall have remedie.

By me, THOMAS LUFFKIN.

Unto this divell incarnate, resorted all sortes of

vayne and undiscrete persons, as it were to a God, to knowe all secretes, paste and to come, specially women, to know how manie husbandes and children they shoulde have, and whether they shoulde burie their husbandes then lyving.   And to be brefe, there was not so great a secrete, that he would not take upon him to declare, unto some he prophecied death within a moneth, who thankes be to God are yet lyving, and in healthe.   All this he boasted that he could do by astronomie ; but when he was talked with of one that had but a yonge and smalle skyll in that arte, he coulde make no directe answere no more then puppe my dogge.

This vilayne coulde wyth a wodden face, bragge, face, and set oute his maters wyth boulde talke, that the symple people was by him mervelously seduced to beleve his lies, and boastinge tales.

Amonge manye that talked with him, one of mine acquaintance asked him this question: Sir, quod he, if you be so cunnynge as ye are named, or as you woulde fayne be estemed to be, wherefore goe ye, and travaile ye from place to place ? for beinge so cunning, ye can not lacke wheresoever ye dwell, for people will resorte unto you farre and nere, sekynge upon you, so that you shoulde not neede thus to travaile for your livynge. Unto whom he made thys beastlye answere ; I knowe, quod he, by astronomye the influence of the starres, and therby perceave when, and howe long any place shall be unto me fortunate, and when I perceave by the starres that any evell fortune is like to chaunce to me in that place, I streighte waye wiselye avoid the daunger, and goe to an other place, wheras I knowe it wil be fortunate and luckye. For what use they to cloke theyr vilanies wyth but astronomye, phisicke, and chirurgery, as I shewed you before.

But thys false knave had answered more truelye if he had sayd thus: though for a tyme as all newe fangels are highlye sette by and mervailed at amonge the folishe and rude people, so naughtye false merchantes, wyth their craftye, and vilainous deseightes, maye for a time have credite and successe according to theyr wicked expectations; yet in a whyle wyth use, the people will begin to smell oute, and be werye of theyr doynges, whiche they at the fyrste so gredelye did seeke, for the strange newes. For suche false deceavers perceave and knowe that the fonde myndes of the common rude multytude of people, at the fyrste, in seekynge to see straunge thynges, are madde of desire, and as they are unreasonable in seekynge the newes, so are they sone werye of the use therof; for muche familiaritye engendereth contempte, even in good thinges; therfore when men begin to perceave and to espye the crafte and subtilty of suche deceavers, it is time for them to change their place, that they maye the easilyer deceave agayne, where theyr falshode is strange and newe, and all together unknowne. If I saye he hadde thus answered, he hadde sayde the very truthe. Thys deceaver hadde sufficiente audacitye, wyth talke to sette oute hys falshode, and to beare downe all that be ignorante, so longe as his knaverye knackes were

unknowne; well, the ende of hys being there, was as
it is common wyth them all, wythoute anye difference,
for he sodainlye was gone wyth manye a poore mannes
monye, whyche he had taken before hande, promisinge
them helpe, whiche onlye he recompensed wyth the
winge of his heles.

Fourthlye, in the yeare of our Lorde a thousande
fyve hundred and three score, one Valentyne came
into a paryshe in the welde of Kente, called Staplehurste; wheras he changed hys name, callynge hym
selfe master Wynkfylde, affirmynge hym selfe to be the
sonne of a worshipful knight of that name. Thys
abhominable deceaver made the people beleve that he
could tel all thinges present, past, and to come; and
the very thoughtes of men, and theyr diseases, by onlye
lokinge in theyr faces. When anye came to hym wyth
urines (whyche commanlye in the countrye they bring
in a stone cruse), he made them beleve that onelye by
feling the weight therof, he would tell them all theyr
diseases in their bodies, or wythout; and otherwhile
made them beleve that he wente to aske councel of the
devel, by going a litle asyde and mumblyng to him
selfe, and then comming agayne, would tell them all,
and more to; for what care of shame or evell have
these hell houndes who see theyr abhomination? but
even as the ape tourneth his filthye partes to every
mannes syghte, so shame they not to acknowledge
them selves to have conference with the divell, that so
yet all wyse men may know theyr dedes to be all divell-
ish, wherin the vaine opinion of some (though not of

the wysest sort), helpeth them not a litle, who esteme
those dampnable artes to be hygh poyntes of learnyng.
Oh ethnike madnesse !

Thys beastlye beguyler so incensed in shorte space
the vayn myndes of the rude and waverynge multitude
of people, that he was sought unto, and estemed more
a greate deale then God, (oh heathenish and idolatrous
people ! not much unlyke this was their outragious
madnes to their pevysh pilgrimages, wherwith in times
past they were most miserably bewiched).   Yea suche
a wonderfull fame and brute wente abroad of his doynges, that some of the verie worshipfulles of those
partes were striken with admiracion, and desyre to
seke to him, to knowe manie good morowes ; wherof
also he would not a lytle bragge and boaste.

But as tyme revealeth all thynges, so this devylyshe
beaste in short tyme was knowne in his righte kynde
and name ; and that he had iii. wyves lyving at that
present, of which the fyrste lyved very porelye and
myserably in Canturbury ; the second, after she knewe
his wickednes, departed from him, and maried after
with a preste ; the third, whiche he at that present
had, he maried at Westmynster, as I was credible in-
formed, beyng there a riche widowe.   But nowe after
this vylaynie was knowne, by his fyrst wyfe comming
to Staplehurste, he ran awaye from hyr also, leavynge
her desolate, undone, and in muche miserie, for he had
spent all her substaunce by riotous fare ; for he was
reported to fare at his table lyke a lorde, and was
served as fynelye as a prynce ; but suche shamefull

dedes can never be withoute wicked ende, at the leaste at Gods hande, thoughe it be neglected of the magistrates.

This laste wyfe beyng sente on his errande to Maydstone, to an apothicaries wydowe for certeyne drougges, chaunced to forgette some of their names, wherewith the women beyng bothe not a lytle troubled, the apothecaries widowe asked whye her husbande dydde not wryte for hys thynges, wherunto his womanne answered that Mayster Wynkfylde was a ryght Latynist, for he coulde wryte no Englyshe.   By this ye maye perceave he was a well learned manne.

This woman beyng as I saide, lefte desolate, maried after with one Thomas Riden, who was his man, who wente together to Westminster, there to dwell, whither not lang after, this Winkefield came, minding agayn to seduce the woman to folowe hym, as before she had ; who so detested his late beastly usance, that she complayned him so to the archebyshop of Canturbury, and other of the quenes majesties honorable councell, that he was long imprysoned in the gate house, and for his wickednes sore punyshed.*   Yet in the ende beynge delyvered, he ceased not any whit to use his olde practise, for he came immediately to Robardesbridge, in Sussexe, where he wrought the lyke wickednesse as afore, and beyng there espied, within a whyle with divers wycked factes, he removed, putting on a brasen face, and came again into Kente, to Staplehurst, wher

---

* He was whipped.

he freshly renewed the use of his odiouse feates, for
the which maister Bissey, person of Staplehurste, caused
him to be ascited of the ordinary to the spirituall courte,
as an adulterer, and a woorker by divlishe and magi-
call artes.   Wherfore he removed two myles from
thence, to a paryshe called Marden, thynkinge him
selfe therby the more salfe, but the lawe notwithstanding, proceded so against him, that he was ther upon
his contempte, excommunicated; and yet never lefte
his olde fashions.   He spent in his house weekely sixe
pound (as dyverse honeste menne reported), in meate
and drynke, with suche resorte and banketyngee, as it
was a wonder to see, whereby he not a litle augmented
his fame ; the people resorting to him farre and nyghe,
for he woulde tell them suche wonders, that all had
hym in admiration.   But especially, he was cunnyng
to inchaunte women to love, and did for rewardes,
dyverse feates in suche cases ; and lastly, he began to
worke properly for himself as foloweth :
    At a paryshe called Loose, in the hundred of Mayd-
stone, a certayne blynde man, called blynde Orgar,
hadde a wyfe who was sycke of dyvers aches and
swellynges, who hearyng of this marveilous monster,
sente hir daughter upon a Wednesday, downe to Marden, with hir water, to this maister Wynkfelde, who
so inchaunted hir, that she forgate hyr waye home to
hyr father and mother in so much that hyr mother
thoughte hyr loste, for she taried there tyll the Satur-
daye folowyng : then takynge hyr waye homewarde,
and beyng come halfe waye, hyr mynde was so intox-

icate, that she retourned backe agayne to hyr lover;
who lovyngly (fearynge leaste hyr frendes shoulde
make exclamation therof), accompanied hir, tyll she was
nyghe at home, and then returning, he promysed hyr
to come to hir mother by a certayne daye, whiche he
in deede performed; and so fylled he the symple woman with suche flatteryng and craftie perswasions, and
fayre promyses of healthe, that she thoughte nothynge
to whotte or to heavy for hym, no, not hyr daughter,
as it apeared, for he forsoke Marden (where he was
xii. pounde in debte, and upwarde), and came to inha-
bite at Loose, in this poore blynde mans house, in so
muche that in a whyle, all people theraboute spake
muche shame, that it was suffered.

The whiche reporte, at suche tyme as it came to the
eares of the worshipfull justices thereaboutes, with also
the trade of his former lyfe, the complaynte of dyverse
honest men whose money he had taken, and deceaved
them: and the clamour of his creditours, to whom he
ought, as is aforesayd.   They sent out their war-
rante, to all constables of that hundred, chargynge
them to aprehende and brynge hym before them at
Maydstone, the Thursdaye folowyng.   Who beynge
warned therof by certeyne disemblyng men, and chiefly
a flatteryng minister, he fledde, and coulde not be
founde, neyther was he synce heard of in that coun-
trey.   This later fitte chanced in the yere of our Lorde
1562, in Lent.   Many more particuler histories coulde
I here wryte of his detestable factes, but to avoyde
prolixity, I leave them at this tyme, trustyng that this

may suffyce to describe what he is, and to geve al men warning of hym and all other lyke deceivers.

The truthe was so ; he had no learnyng in the world, nor coulde reade Englishe (and, as I suppose, knewe not a letter, or a b from a bateldore), as it was well proued, yet made he the people beleve that he coulde speake Latin, Greek, and Hebrue.

Item in the yere 1562, there came to the towne of Maidstone an olde felowe, who tooke upon him to heale all diseases, as a profounde phisitien, whom (for be- cause men had been so deluded by divers former de- ceivers,) I caused to be examined before the officers of the said towne.   And when he was asked his name, he said, John Bewly ; secondly, wher he dwelte, and he answered at London, in the Old Bayly, against Sir Roger Chamley.   Thirdly, if he were a phisitien, he sayde yea.   Fourthly, where he learned that arte, and he sayde by his owne study.   Fiftly, where he studied it, he answered, in his owne house.   Sixtly, what authours he had redde, he sayde, Eliote, and others.   Seventhly, we asked what other, and he said, he had forgotten.   Eightly, we asked him what weare the names of Eliotes bookes, he sayd, he re- membered not.   Then we brought him an Englyshe booke to reade, whiche he refused ; but when he was commaunded to rede, he desired us to be good to him, for he was a poore man, and in deede coulde not reade, and sayd that he intended not to tary there, but to re- payre home agayne.   This beyng done on a Sondaye, after evensong, his hoste was bounde for his foorthcomming the next daie, when upon his humble sute, he was let goe; beyng warned with exhortations, to leave suche false and naughty deceytes.

Farther in the same yere, one William, a shomaker, came into Kente, pretending to be very cunning in curing diseases of the eyes; and being brought to a frende of myne, to have his judgement in ones eye, whereof the sight was weake; first putting them in muche feare of the eye, he at lengthe promised to doe great thinges therto.   But the frendes of the partie diseased desired me first to talke with him, to understande his cunning; which I, at their request, did, at a tyme appointed, and asked him if he understoode what was the cause of hir infirmitie.   He said he could not tel, but he wold heale it he doubted not.   Then I asked him whether he were a surgien, or a phisitien; and he answered, no, he was a shomaker, but he coulde heale all maner of sore eyes.

I asked him where he learned that; he sayde that was no matter.   Well, sayde I, seyng that you can heale sore eyes, what is an eye? whereof is it made? of what members or partes is it composed? and he sayde he knewe not that.

Then I asked hym if he weare worthy to be a shoemaker, or to be so called, that knewe not howe, or wherof a shoe was made? he answered no, he was not worthy.   Then, sayde I, how dare you worke upon suche a precious and intricate member of man as is the eye, seyng you knowe not the nature therof? and why, or by what reason, it doth see more then a mans nose,

c

or his hand dothe ?   He answered, that though he could
not tell this, yet could he heale all maner of sore eyes.
And that where as maister Luke of London, hath a
great name of curyng eyes, he coulde doe that which
maister Luke could not doe, nor turne his hande to.
Thus bragged this proude varlette, against and above
that reverent man of knowne learning and experience.

And I sayde I thought so, for Maister Luke, sayde
I, is no shoemaker. Well, sayde he, I perceive you doe
but skorne me, and flunge out of the doores in a great
fume, and coulde not be caused to tary and drynke by
any intreaty, neither have I since that tyme heard any
thyng of hym.

What other men and women, besydes these, have
come into the forsayde place, if I should rehearse them,
and the discourse of their doinges, it weare to tedious,
yea, it wold abhorre any honest mans eares to heare
of it.   There came a woman thither, (as she reported
hirself), a ministers wife, (but I thynke she falsely
lyed), in the aforesayde yeare. The officers hearing
of hir prophession, called hir before them, and examined hir, with whom she was so stoute, as to say
(when she was warned to departe the towne, in payne
of imprysonment), these wordes: I have, quod she,
travelled through all partes of this realme, and I was never yet forbidden in any place to minister my physike,
and hath (sayde she), your towne a privilege above
all other, to forbydde me to doe good, and to heale the
queenes leige people ? Then was she asked what authoritie she hadde, or of whom she was allowed thus to

dooe, or what certificat she hadde brought with hir, to witnes with hir of hir good behavour in places where she was before? and she sayde she was never before so examined, neither feared to be put to suche triall, neither sawe she ever the place, that a woman coulde fynde so little curtesie, especially sithe she asked no-thynge gratis of any man, or otherwyse then for hir mony: these stoute wordes notwithstanding, she was expelled the towne.

And not longe after, came thither a make shifte, with two men wayghting on hym, as very rakehelles as him selfe, bragging that he was a profounde phisicien ; and being called by the officers to examination, was so streyghtly charged, that he confessed himselfe and his men, to be felowes in frendshippe, and all of one krewe ; and this was a shifte, mutually devised among them to get mony ; and so weare they expelled the towne ; or rather they shifted sodainly away for feare of punyshement ; whiche if they had taried, they could not have escaped, so good then was the mynde of the officers for that yeare.   And now one historie of the tyme present, to knitte up this my tale of vagabondes and rennegates most hatefull.

One Robert Nicols, a false deceiver, and moste igno-raunt beaste, and of the profession of vagaboundes, (as weare his former felowes), hath in tymes passed boasted him selfe to have been the servaunt of Maister Vicary, late sargeant chyrurgien to the queenes highnes.   But now the matter being put in triall, he sayeth he was apprentice with a priest, among whose wicked and pro-

digious doynges, (whiche are infinite, one very notable
chaunced in the yere of our Lorde 1564, the 26 of
September; he poured in a purgation to an honest
woman of good fame, one Riches, wydowe, of Linton,
(a paryshe of three myles distant from Maydestone),
whiche within three or foure houres at the moste,
purged the lyfe out of hir body, so violent was this
mortal potion. The woman being before in perfecte
health, to all mens judgementes, beinge onely of sim-
plicitie perswaded to take the same, by the deceivable
perswasions of this Nicols, who made fayre wether of
all thynges, and hir to beleve that he would deliver hir
of suche diseases as in deede she had not. For he
should have had by composition, xx. shillinges for the
saide drynke.

For this murderous facte, he was by the queenes
majesties justices apprehended, and imprisoned in the
gaile of Maydstone, where he was communed with all,
concernyng his knowledge and doynges, and for what
cause he gave hir that purgation, and howe she was
perswaded to take it. He answered, that he knewe
by hir complexion, that hyr lyver and hyr lunges weare
rotten, and therfore he toulde hyr so. Wherunto one
replyed sayinge, naye, she was not sycke, but thou tould-
est hyr so for thy fylthye lucre, and she beleved thee.
And because (as thou saydest), thou knewest all this
by hyr complexion, I praye thee what complexion am
I of ? He answered, you are sanguine.

Then was it asked him, whether it weare proper to
a sanguine man to have blacke heare, as that partye

hadde on his bearde? to this he answered, O, ye wyll
saye ye are more a the choler. Then the partie gave
hym hys hande to feele, which was commonly colde,
saiynge, is a cholericke man wonte to be so colde?
whiche when he hadde felte, he sayde : O then ye
woulde be of the fleme. Then was he asked, what is
a sanguine man? or why is he called sanguine? he
answered, a sanguine man is he that hathe a good dis-
gesture. Mary, as thou sayest, quod the demaunder,
here in hast thou shewed howe great thy cunnynge
is in judgyng complexions. Then was it saide to hym,
ye professe bothe phisicke and chirurgerie, what authours have you redde? He answered, Vigo and
Gasken.

Then was it demaunded, what medicyne gavest thou
the woman wherwith thou haddeste so evyll lucke?
And he sayde, *catapussis*. Then beynge rebuked for
that he would take on hym to geve medicyne inwardlye,
whereof he knewe not the names, muche lesse the
nature : he sayde as stoutely, as obstinatly, that he
knewe as many purgations as the partie that reproved
hym. Then he asked hym of foure or five, such as
came first to minde, as tamar indes, mirobalanes, aga-
rick, &c., of all the whiche he sayd he knew none.
Then was he requyred to name them that he dyd know,
and he sayde he knewe *catapussis*, and *catapistela*.

Then was he asked what *catapistela* was. Why,
quod he to the demaunder, doe not you knowe it?
No, sayde the partie, not by that name. And it was
further asked whether it weare an herbe, a roote, a

tree, a stone, the hove, horne, or tayle of a beaste, or what it was? Nicols answered that it was none of those, but a thynge made beyonde the seas. It is not made in Englande, quod he, I thynke it be made in Fraunce. Then was he agayne reproved for his beastly braggyng. And here maiest thou see, quod the person that reasoned with hym, thyne owne ignoraunce, in that thou sayest it is made, wher it is in deed the fructe of a tree called *cassia fistula*, (as I thynke thou meanest), and not *catapistela*. And he answered, (not withstandyng his former impudencie), it is so; saiyng also thus, oh, you call it *casia*, belyke because it is lyke a case.

Then this man begynning to prove his cunnyng in the natures of symples, asked hym the nature of peper. He sayde it was hotte in the firste degree, and colde in the seconde. Why then, sayde the demaundaunt, what saye you to the nature of an oyster? and he, (answerynge as before of the temperamente), sayde colde in the fyrst degree, and hotte in the thyrde. Then was it sayde to the standers by, here may you see his beastly ignorance, dyd ye ever heare that two contraries coulde dwelle together and agree in one subjecte? Wherunto this lewde felowe most proudly answered, though I can not reason so well as you, but am confounded at your hande, yet have I done great and many cures, whiche, sayd he, commeth of somewhat, though you saye I knowe nothyng. After this, one asked him if he weare by authoritie admitted, accordinge to the lawes of this realme, to use phisicke and chirurgery, as a practiser of the same? To whom

an other sayde; thynke you that any such ignorant
asse as this is, can be any where so admitted?   Unto
all this he sayde, if none should be suffered to use them
but the learned, or suche as are permitted, a great
manye poore people should perishe for lacke of helpe.
To this he was answered, nay, rather a great numbre
that are daily kylled or lamed, by suche ignorant
beastes as thou arte, might, (by the benefite of nature,
and other good helpes of cunnyng men), recover right
well, and lyve, if suche as thou art weare not.

Among other questions of the anatomie, to al the
which he answered as beastly as in other thinges before.
It was asked him what the splene was, and he answered,
that it was a disease in the syde, baked hard lyke a
bisket; deniyng that there was any thyng called the
splene, but the disease, (sayeth he), so called.

Then was it further demaunded of him, (because he
boasted muche of chirurgerie), what a wounde was;
and he answered, a wounde is a hurte, or a bruse.
What is an ulcer, then, sayde the opponente? he answered, an ulcer is a wounde.   And then beyng asked
whether a wounde and an ulcer weare all one, he sayde,
a wounde is that whiche is newe, and an ulcer is that
whiche is olde.   To this it was replied, that an ulcer
might also be newe, and that it was an ulcer though it
weare but one daye olde.   After this he sayde that he
knewe an ulcer with a canker, also a marmole and a
fistula.   Wherfore he was asked what was a canker,
and he sayde, a canker is when an ulcer doth by rankling become a canker.   Wherunto one replied, saying,

a cancer may in dede be ulcerate, and is often so; but
that every ulcer may by rankling (as thou saiest) become a cancer, it hath not been redde nor seen.   But
then he sayde that he spake of a canker, and not of a
cancer; for a cancer, sayde he, is when an ulcer
stynketh.

Muche more could I wryte of his beastly answeres,
if I thought this not enough, yea, to much, except it
weare better.   And though I thinke this enough to
greve any wyse mans eyes to see, or eares to heare,
yet shall I desyre them to beare with a worde or twayne
more, that what they are, even the unskilfull may perceive, and learne to beware of them.

A certaine pacient of myne, (having lately been
cured at my hande), metynge with this Nicols at his
brothers house, reasoned with hym of a payne that he
sometyme hadde in his hyppe; I trowe, quod he, ye
cal it a sciatica, doe ye not?   Yea, sayde Nicols, there
is a sciatica, and a sciitica.   Then sayde my pacient, I
never hearde my chyrurgien name any suche.   Who
is that, sayde Nicols? and my pacient named me.
Then began Nicols to praise a neighbour of myne, saiyng that he was cunninger then I, but my pacient
praysed me to be cunninger then my neighbour.   Yea,
sayd Nicols, in talke, Halle can talke better.   Then
sayde my paciente, I hadde a grevous sore legge, with
greate apostemacions and hollownes, wherefore if he
coulde have done nothing but talke, he myght have
talked long enough to my legge before it would so have
been whole.

Unto the same man also he made his vaunte
on a a tyme, that he sawe his maister, close a mans
head together, that was clefte from the crowne of the
head, down to the necke, who sayde he was after healed,
and did live.   This shamles lye, beyng hearde of a mery
man, was with an other like lye quited, on this sorte.
Tushe, (sayd this mery man), I have heard of as great
a matter as this; for a certayne man fallyng into the
handes of theves, was robbed, and his head was so
smoothe cutte off, that it stoode styll upon his necke
tyll he rode home; whose wyfe metyng hym at the
doore, perceived his bosome bloudy, and asked hym if
hys nose had bledde; whiche wordes when the man
hearde, he tooke his nose in his hand to blowe it, and
therwith threw his head in at the dore.   And nowe as
it is tyme I leave also this monster, least I should to
muche weary the lovynge reader, with the long readyng
of these moste frivolous communications, and tragedi-
ous doynges, (which I have with griefe of harte written, trusting that it will not onely be a warning unto
some, that they committe not their lyfe and healthe in
sicknesse, unto suche lyfe purgers, but also that in commyng to the handes of some vertuous menne, may
with the pitie of other mens myseries, move them to
laboure, to the most of their power, to redresse these
evels).   Omitting also one Carter, otherwyse called
Carvell, otherwyse Maye, who is a sorcerer, and a
worker by dyvelyshe spirites, clokyng the same under
the colour of phisick, and hath done much mischief
among the people, with his abhorrefull doynges, whiche

I will hereafter (as leysoure and occasion shall serve), farther declare.

I will here also omitte to talke of Grigge the poulter, with divers other, whose endes have made their doinges knowne. And also of a joyner in London, a Frencheman borne, that is of late becomme a phisitien, who is estemed at this daye, among dyverse ryght worshipfull, to be very learned and cunnyng, that knowe not his originall; yea, they call him doctor James; but an honest woman, an olde neighbour of his, (not longe synce), at a man of worshyppes house in Kente, merveyled to see hym in suche braverye, and lordly apparell; who, when she tooke acquaintance of hym, he wronge hyr harde by the hande, and rounded hyr in the eare, saiyng: if thou be an honest woman, kepe thy tongue in thy headde, and saye nothinge of me.

For surely a monstrous great legende should I make, if I shoulde here recite all suche, as I have knowne and heard of; but if any man would knowe more of the doynges of these deceyvers and runnegates, let hym reade a little booke called a Galley late come into Englande, from Terra Nova, laden with Phisitiens, Apothecaries, and Chirurgiens, &c., the author wherof I knowe not. Also let them reade a little worke, entituled, A Poesie, made in forme of a vision, &c., lately imprinted. Also let them reade the verses of maister Bulleyne, in his Bulwarke, in the dialogue betwene sorenes, and chirurgery; where he ryghte truly and pleasantly describeth them in their ryght colours. In the whiche boke also in divers places, he noteth the sleighty practises of suche abusers as he hath knowne in divers countries.

What shall we thinke Diogenes would saye, if he now lived, and sawe so many rusticall craftesmen leave their misteries, and become phisitiens? seynge he sayde to one that was a weake wrestler, (and after became a phisitien), these wordes in effecte: what intendest thou nowe, quod he, craftily and privily be revenged of them that weare wont to vanquishe or overthrowe thee? Or what would Socrates nowe saye, who saide (upon like occasion), to a paynter that became a phisitien; nowe thou workest subtillye, (quod he), for wheras before thyne errors were espied, and judged of all men, nowe thou wylt hyde them in the earth, or bury them in the ground. Meanyng (without doubt), that such phisiciens are more like to kil men, than to save or heale them.

Well sure if there were good orders in all places, and the holesome lawes of this realme well executed, there coulde none such deceyve, with theyr running about, and kreping into corners, unsuspected, and examined. For it is easy to conjecture, or rather perfectlye to knowe, that no honest cunning man, that meaneth trulye and justlye, will refuse to dwell and continue in some estemed city or towne, (for unto such wise and learned men delight to resort), and to run about here and there, through all the realme, thus like vacaboundes, to deceive the unskilfull people wyth theyr beastly doinges.

I trust yet one day to see it better loked on : and in
the meane season, let a great many abusers (whome I
knowe, especially in Kent, bothe men and women, and
have not here named them), repent and leve their
wickednes, otherwise let them assure them selves I wil
no more stay to publysh them with their wicked
doings, and knavery knackes, bringing them into this
register, then I have don to set forth these.

It shall behove every good chirurgien therfore, to
place hym selfe in some good towne, or famous citye,
and surelye the people will resort unto hym, and send
for him at theyr nede, to hys sufficient profit and liv-
ing ; neither wyll anye good man despeyre of thys.

It can not be without suspicion therfore, either of
the lacke of cunnyng, or of a deceivable false con-
science, that a chirurgien, or phisitien, shall refuse to
fixe himselfe constantly in some dwellyng place, and
to become a wanderynge fugitive, as these were and
are, of whom I have wrytten.

Notwithstanding, I am not ignorant that constante
dwellers may be also deceavyng abusers, so long as ther
is no punyshment, nor execution of lawes to the contrary, as for example.

One named Kiterell, dwelleth in Kente, at a parysh
called Bedersden, that hath been all his lyfe a sawyer
of tymber and borde, a man very symple, and altogether unlearned ; who at this present is become a phisitien, or rather a detestable deceavyng sorcerer.   He
wyll geve judgement on urines, and whyles he loketh
on the water, he will grope and fele him selfe all about ;

and otherwhyle, where as he feleth, he will shrynke, as
though he were pricked, or felte some great paine.
Then he tourneth to the messenger and telleth him
where, and in what sorte the partie is greved; whiche
maketh the people thynke him very cunning.   They
seeke to hym farre and neere for remedy for suche as
are bewyched or inchanted, and as they commonly
terme it, forespoken.   What stuffe is this, let the wyse
and learned judge.   And he hath so prospered with
these doynges, that in shorte space he hath been able
bothe to purchase and buylde, as I am credibly enformed of divers men that doe knowe and have seen the
same.   For there are many that reporte, (and they no
small fooles,) that he hath cured suche as al the learned
phisitiens in England coulde doe no good unto, beleve
it who wyll.

Notwithstanding Cardanus, a learned philosopher,
in his worke *De Subtilitate*, in the tenthe booke therof,
intituled of spirites or divels, seemeth to prove that
there are certayne griefes, chaunsing sometime to mans
body by enchauntement, or the workyng of cursed
sciences; wherof for so muche as phisicke and chirurgerie knowe no cause, they are also to seeke of a remedy.   For in these laudable artes, there is a reasonable cause founde of every disease, upon the reason
wherof, ther is ordeined a remedy.   But when through
divilyshe and wicked sciences there is any sycknesse
procured, wherof the laudable arte of medicine knoweth not the cause, so can it procure no helpe, but only
by helpe of some of those sciences most detestable,

must the same be taken away agayne ; so that it seemeth to be a common composition among them, the one
to tormente the bodies both of man and beastes, that
an other may be sought unto to remedy the same. So
one beyng ever a workynge instrument to an other.

It may chance nowe that some whose myndes are
already affectionate to those artes, will saye, that it is
necessary that such men should be, for the comforte of
them that have neede, when as no helpe otherwise wil
serve.   To whom it may be answered, that if they be
Christian men, they ought not to seke helpe at divels,
sithe the Holy Ghost, by the mouth of Sayncte Paule,
hath warned, that no man doe evell that good may come
therof.   Farthermore, if none suche (as God in his
holy lawe hath commaunded), were suffred to lyve,
there could no such inconvenience chaunce, wherby
any man should have neede to seke to them for helpe,
seynge that there is never any neede of their ayde,
but where the effect is firste caused, through the wycked
workyng of those damnable artes.   But let this suffice
that we have spoken, concernyng the wycked abuses of
phisicke and chirurgerie, and lette us nowe procede to
the dutie of the chirurgien, and the good observation
of his office, whiche wyll avoyde these, and all lyke
abuses, wherunto at this day (God amende it), phisicke
and chyrurgery is made a cloke.   For none of these
false merchantes wyll wyllyngly be called by the name
of that whiche they moste use, but they wyll be called
phisiciens, chirurgiens, and astronomers, when they can
as muche skyll in any of them as brute beastes.

And concernynge the behavour that is requyred in a true chirurgien to his paciente, and of one chirurgien to an other concernynge councell, honeste workyng, and knowledge, I have thought good to gather the councels, and good documentes of dyvers good and veterate authores, (and have formed the same into Englyshe verses, or metre), and here to place the same, for the better instruction of all yonge chirurgiens, that it may as well be easy to learne, as apte to be kepte in memorie, of all wyllynge learners.

HARKE, and drawe nere, ye younge studentes,
　　Your eares loke ye unclose ;
The worthye arte chirurgery,
　　To practise that purpose.

And marke what the greate masters saye,
　　That here before have wroughte ;
And did to theyr disciples leave,
　　In wrytinge what they taughte.

And to theyr scholers did descrive,
　　A briefe methode or waye ;
Commaundinge them the same to marke,
　　On thys wise gan they saye : —

When thou arte callde at anye time,
　　A patient to see ;
And doste perceave the cure to greate,
　　And ponderous for thee :

See that thou laye disdeyne aside,
　　And pride of thyne owne skyll:
And thinke no shame counsell to take,
　　But rather wyth good wyll

Gette one or two of experte men,
　　To helpe thee in that nede;
And make them partakers wyth thee,
　　In that worke to procede.

For in so doinge, thine honestye
　　Thou shalte well kepe and save;
Also thy patiente therby
　　Righte greate comforte shall have.

By thys meanes thou mayste haplye learne,
　　Ryghte seldome sene before;
Of thee, or hym, whyche fyrste thee taughte,
　　Thoughe thou have cunnynge store.

And also if oughte goe a wrye,
　　Or hinder in thy cure,
The one maye mende the others faulte,
　　While frendship dothe endure.

The wounded or sore man also,
　　Shall have no cause to grudge
In you suche uniformitye,
　　Whyle he maye see and judge.

And farthermore thou haste thy parte,
  Bothe of profyt and fame ;
When that your worke hathe good successe,
  And luckilye dothe frame.

And if it happe to frame amisse,
  Suspicyon can be none ;
Sythe thou haste soughte all meanes of healthe,
  And wouldste not be alone.

So eche man shall with other beare,
  Thy juste cause to defende ;
All wise and learned men also,
  Shall thee prayse and commende.

For all that be discrete doubtlesse,
  Wyll judge thee to be wyse ;
In that thou doest desyre to learne,
  And augmente thy practise.

And wylte not that throughe negligence,
  And pride of thine owne waye ;
Thy pacient in paine shoulde spill,
  To perishe and dekaye.

Thy purpose thus thou shalte attaine,
  Wyth ease and honestye ;
Where otherwyse it maye thee brynge,
  Shame and ignominye.

D

And farther if thou waye it righte,
　　It is easie to gesse ;
That better two, then one alone,
　　All errores maye redresse.

For as all men that here doe live,
　　Borne in this wretched vale,
Are fraughted full of errores greate,
　　Oure boote mixed wyth bale ;

From whyche the prudent Salomon,
　　Was never voide and free ;
As of him selfe he wryteth playne,
　　Who so will reade maye see.

So if thou in chirurgerye,
　　Alone wylte walke and wade ;
Thine errores will thy worke confounde,
　　And all thine honoure quade.

Sithe Bernarde* knewe not all hym selfe,
　　Thinke never in thy minde ;
But that at laste by painfull proofe,
　　Thou shalt thine errores fynde.

For errores, not staide at the firste,
　　But suffred to procede,

---

* This is an allusion to Lanfranc's " Chirurgia Parva," which
was addressed to his pupil Bernard.

To mischiefes greate, as Plato saythe,
   Will growe in verye dede.

But the beginninge if thou stoppe,
   By good counsell and pure;
All doubtfull thynges thou shalt prevent,
   And harde diseases cure.

For all to late comes remedye,
   When throughe thy negligence
The griefe is growne paste aide and cure,
   And all experience.

But one thinge note, when two or moe
   Together joygned be;
Aboute the paynfull patient,
   See that ye doe agree.

See that no discorde doe arise,
   Nor be at no debate;
For that shall sore discomforte hym,
   That is in sycke estate.

And when alone with your foreman,
   One of you is presente;
Defame nor dispraise in no wise,
   The same that is absente.

For noughte can more discomforte him,
   That lies in griefe and peyne,

Then heare that one of you dothe beare,
  To other suche disdeine.

Wherfore what so ye have to saye,
  In thinges aboute your arte ;
Let it be done among your selves,
  In secrete and a parte.

Wyth one consent uniformlye
  Comforte the wounded man ;
But unto some good frende of hys
  Expresse all that ye can.

And let them knowe the daunger greate,
  That like is to succede ;
Prognosticatinge wittilye,
  And in convenient spede.

Wherfore eche one of you shall take,
  At other his counsell,
Howe that in moste convenient wise,
  Ye may the griefe expell.

And so that one in anye wise,
  From other nothinge hide ;
But by all meanes consulte, and for
  The sicke mannes healthe provide.

For in that nede if any doe
  His counsell kepe a loofe,

And so the wounded man decaye,
    It shall be his reproofe.

See that for goulde or covetise,
    Ye take no thing in hande,
Whiche incurable for to be,
    Ye doe well understand.

Or oughte unlesse to cure the same
    Thou have some perfecte grounde ;
For if thou doe, it will thy fame
    In utter shame confounde.

Looke of thy selfe in anye wise,
    Thou make no praise nor boste ;
For that shall turne to thy dispraise,
    When thou doest use it moste.

See thou dispraise none other man,
    His error thoughe thou knowe ;
For sure an other for thy plage,
    Shall thee like curtsye showe.

Commende the dedes of eche good man,
    The best loke that thou saye ;
So shall good fame redounde to thee,
    From all men day by daye.

Not onlye in chirurgery,
    Thou oughtest to be experte ;

But also in astronomye,
   Bothe prevye and aperte.

In naturall philosophye,
   Thy studye shoulde be bente ;
To knowe eche herbe, shrubbe, roote, and tree,
   Muste be thy good intente.

Eche beaste and foule, wyth worme and fishe,
   And all that beareth lyfe ;
Their vertues and their natures bothe,
   With thee oughte to be rife.

And in the grounde metall and stone,
   And veines of earthe also ;
Their powres and vertues in degre,
   Shoulde not be hid the fro.

But chieflye the anatomye,
   Ye ought to understande ;
If ye will cure well anye thinge,
   That ye doe take in hande.

For by the same above the rest,
   Ye shall greate fame deserve ;
The life of man from manye streightes,
   To save and well preserve.

Withoute the knowledge of whyche arte,
   Thou canste not chose but erre ;

In all that thou shalte goe aboute,
   Thy knowledge to preferre.

As if ye cutte or cauterize,
   Or use phlebotomye ;
Ye can not but erre in the same,
   Withoute anatomye.

He is no true chirurgien,
   That can not shewe by arte,
The nature of evrye member,
   Eche from other aparte.

For in that noble handye worke,
   There dothe nothinge excell
The knowledge of anatomye,
   If it be learned well.

Endevoure therfore by all meanes,
   The same to know and cunne,
For when thou haste it perfectlye,
   Thine arte is halflye wunne.

For therby shalt thou understande,
   Of eche member in dede,
Their nature and their offices,
   And howe they doe procede.

And unto what good use they serve,
   As well the leaste as moste ;

And by their hurte prognosticate
What action will be loste.

Wherby of knowledge and greate skill,
  Thou shalt obteine the brute;
And men to thee in generall,
  For helpe shall make their sute.

Wherfore all honour, laude, and praise,
  To God ascribed be;
The Father, Sonne, and Holye Ghoste,
  One God and personnes three.

Perhappes nowe some man wyll object and saye, that
it is not possible alwayes to observe these rules.   For
if I dwell farre from expert men of whome to aske
councell, and peradventure am matched in the place
where I dwell, with some braggynge proud boye, that
came latelye oute of his prentishode, who shall for
lacke of knowledge and discretion seke myne infamy
and dishonour, and is therfore not mete to associate my
selfe wyth, but rather to be avoided.

To this I answer, that it behoveth a good chirurgien
to be ingenious, and that in this case is thy remedy.
To be ingenious, is to be apte to devise newe remedies
for new diseases, and suche as thou haste not before
seene nor hearde of.

In suche a case in deede it behoveth thee to be verye
polytique, and that Allmightye God maye the better
prosper all thy workes and devises, serve God faith-

fullye in hartye contemplacions daye and nighte, desir-
inge God for Jesus Christes sake, hys dere Sonne oure
Savyoure, to enspire thee wyth suche grace, that thou
maiste to his honor and glory, ende all suche enter-
prises as thou takest upon thee to doe; (of whyche
prayer I will hereafter wryte an example), for if God
be on thy syde, feare not who so ever be agaynst thee.
And that thou mayste the better knowe what thou
doste, that wilt be a chirurgien, and what thou takest
upon thee to professe, knowe oute of good and learned
authores, what chirurgerye is, and so shalte thou be the
better able wiselye to worke alone, where the nedefull
society of counsell dothe wante.

Chirurgery, therefore, (as Angelus Bolognius in the
prologe to his boke of the cure of externall ulcers,
sayeth), is the moste aunciente, ye the moste sure and
excellente parte of the arte of medicyne, whiche worketh by handy operation.   For the name thereof whiche
was geven thereto by moste auncyent authores, signi-
fieth nothynge elsse; for chirurgery is *Operatio Man-
ualis*, that is handye worke.   Wherfore syth it is a
parte of phisike, we can not so rightlye name it in
Englishe, as to call it the handye worke of medicine.
And farthermore the arte of medicine or phisicke,
(wherin chirurgery is comprehended), is an arte, and
so it oughte to be named, and not a science; and chirurgery is not an arte properlye of it selfe wythoute
phisike, or seperated from the same, as some doe thinke;
neyther can phisike be an whole and perfecte arte
wythout chirurgery, as some woulde imagin.   For

sythe they are both partes one of an other, how can
they be devided or separate wythout detriment to
them bothe? for it is not a whole body that lacketh
one of hys chiefe members, or partes; for nether can
chirurgerye be perfectlye learned wythoute theorike,
nor phisike wythoute practise. And wheras theorike
and practise goe not together, whether ye call it phisike or chirurgery, I dare boldlye affirme, that there is
in them no manner of perfection worthy commenda-
tion. Yet some there be that thinke that onlye to
phisike belongeth theorike, or speculation, and that to
chirurgery belongeth onlye practise; but howe farre
their judgementes differ from truthe, let everye wyse
man judge. What knowledge is there in phisike that
is not requisyte in chirurgerye? whether it be gramer,
philosophy, astronomye, anatomye, or anye other; ye,
the very judiciall of urine, and the pulse, as good doctor Record, our worthye countrye man witnesseth;
wherfore I affyrme, accordynge to the sentence of moste
wise authoures, that the knowledge of chirurgerye
consisteth in ii. thinges, namelye, speculation and practise, and therfore it is not only a workinge, but an
excellente knowledge, and understandynge howe to
worke well and perfectly. But the effectuall actes of
chirurgerye in deede, (as Guido saythe), consyste in
cuttinge, in knittinge, in bindinge, in purgyng, purify-
ing, and exercisynge the handye operation, and all this
upon the bodye of man, to heale, or bring health to the
same, as muche as is possible. Whiche addition we
put to, because it never hath ben, is, nor shalbe possi-

ble for any chirurgien to heale all that are diseased and sore. Therfore we maye thus conclude that chirurgery is an arte both workynge and teachinge how to worke upon the bodye of man, to heale all suche diseases as are possible to be cured.

Nowe therfore, let the good chirurgien, (that wil avoyde wicked crafts and abuses), first learne, and then worke and use experience; wherin thou shalt understande that the onlye readinge in bookes is not sufficient, as manye a one at this day, (to the great hurt of muche people), thinketh. For there is no science that can wythoute seinge the practyse and experience of cunnyng masters therin, be lerned; and surelye in the arte of medicine, (chieflye chirurgerye), practise and experience is the chiefest learnyge; although withoute other learnynge (I confesse) no man can attayne to the perfection that therin is required. And for this dothe learnynge (in bookes conteined), chiefly serve to teache men to knowe the workes of learned masters of old tyme; but assure thy selfe, (what so ever suche masters have wrytten), thou shalt never perfectlye digest to thine owne use, anye thinge in them, except thou be able to joyne by comparison, that which thou haste sene in other mennes workes before thine eies, and in the practise of thine owne handes, wyth that whiche thou findest wrytten in olde authors; for lyttle profit, swetenesse, or understandinge shall one gette of authores except he see the same also put in practise. Therfore when thou haste sene proved by cunning masters, the whyche thou haste red, thou arte trulye learned in

thine arte, and therfore apte to worke and use experience thy selfe.

And this regarde to experience in learninge made
Socrates say, that lerning ought not to be wrytten in
bokes, but rather in mennes mindes. For this excellent philosopher well perceived that the committinge
of cunnyng to wrytten bookes, made men to neglect
the practise and experience of their wittes by meanes
wherof they became uncunninge.

Galen also hathe frendly admonished us, that we
ought not, (if we will be perfectlye cunninge), to trust
onelye to doctrine wrytten in bokes, but rather oure
propre eyes, whiche are to be trusted above all other
authores, ye, before Hippocrates and Galen ; for wythout the eyes consent, (saith Socrates), the eares oughte
not to be trusted ; for the eares are subjectes, and often
deceived, but the eyes are judges bothe true and certaine.

As I woulde therfore, that all chirurgiens shoulde
be learned, so woulde I have no man thinke him selfe
lerned otherwise then chiefly by experience ; for learning in chirurgery consisteth not in speculation only,
nor in practise only, but in speculation well practised
by experience. Therfore when we saye that a chirurgien muste firste be learned, and then worke, it is
not ment that any man by the reading of a booke, or
bokes onlye, may learne how to worke, for truelye that
hathe caused so many deseivinge abusers, as there are
at this daye.

Good chirurgien, therfore, have a regard to these

things, even as thou wilte answer for the same at the
dredful daye, when the eternall Lord, and almighty
Master, shall call for accompt of eche mannes talent,
whether they have gained therwith, accordinge to his
will, or whether they have abused, or vainlye hid the
same.

Furthermore, these thinges considered and observed,
it is expedient chiefly, and before all thinges, that thou
have Goddes feare alwaies before thine eies, that thou
leade a vertuous life, and (as nere as God shal geve
thee grace), unspotted to the world, doing just and vertuous dedes, abhorring and abstaining from all vicious-
nesse.   Let wicked pride be farre from thy hart, and
rather with all humility confesse that thou canst doe
nothing of thy selfe, (as thou canste not in deede), but
through the grace and mercifull favoure of God.

Likewise avoide envye and wicked wrathe ; be neyther wrathfull, nor envyous, that an other man of thyne
arte hathe better successe then thy selfe, but rather
endevoure thy self in the feare and service of God, to
learne to doe better, and to excede others.   For to a
diligente and wyllynge minde, there is nothing to harde
ne impossible.

Let charitye surmounte covetise, so that it have no
place in thy harte, otherwise then it shall be requisite
for thee to live like a man of science with a decent and
honest maintenance of necessaryes.   Let no slouthe
cause thee to neglecte thy cures, wherof thou haste
taken charge, least through thy negligence they pear-

ishe, and their bloud call for vengance on thee at the handes of God.

In anye wise be thou no lechoure, but adorne thy life wyth honest, chaste, and sober manners; for that uncleane and filthye vice is muche to be abhorred in a chirurgyen, consideringe the secretes of manye honest folkes, that to hys charge and cure muste be committed.

Lastlye, and above all these, beware of dronkennesse, a vyce that was never more used, then it is of manye at this tyme. For when hathe this vile reporte (or rather reproche), gone of so manye as it dothe at this daye, he is a good chirurgyen in the forenone? O abhomination of all other in a chirurgien to be detested! but how unmete suche arte to be chirurgiens I have touched more at large in my preface.

Let vertue, therfore, I saye, be thy guide; let hir be bothe thy rule and compasse, wherby to frame all thy doinges.

And consider that chirurgerye is an arte to heale dyseases, whyche is a vertuous exercise, ye, a gifte of Goddes spiryte, as saythe S. Paule; and therfore can never be well used of vicious personnes, althoughe they have never so muche lerninge; for vice and vertue can never accorde, but alwayes one is expelled by the other, for two contraries can never agree in one subjecte.

Consider, also, howe by vertuous and holye lyfe, and by faithfull prayer, the very angelles at Goddes appoyntment have descended from heaven to aid and helpe men in their nede, teachinge them remedies for

divers griefes ; as holye Raphaell was sent to Tobye.
And as thou mayste reade in the xxxviii. chapiter of
Jesus, the sonne of Sirache, wher he, (treatinge of the
phisitien), saythe : the houre maye come that the sycke
maye be healed throughe them when they praye unto
the Lorde, that he maye recover and get health to lyve
longer.   Loe, here mayste thou see that thy duety is
to praye unto God for thy pacient, and for helpe and
grace to heale him.   Praye, therefore, faithfully unto
God, serve hym devoutlye, call rightlye upon his holy
name daye and night, wyth an holye abstinence as
scripture teacheth, not omyttinge dedes of almes, the
frutes of perfecte faythe.

   Moreover, be not ingrate nor unthankefull unto God
when he sendeth good successe to thy businesse, good
lucke to thy handes, and graunteth thee thy hartes
desyre.   For unthankfulnesse many times is the cause
that our prayers are not heard.   Praise God, therfore,
for his benefites, and pray faithfullye to hym in all thy
streightes of nede, and this doinge, be sure that God
will prosper all thy wayes, and geve good successe to
all thy workes.   Take here, therefore, an example of
prayer whiche thou mayste use, I trust, to the glorye
of God.

A PRAYER NECESSARYE TO BE SAYDE OF ALL CHIRURGIENS.

O ALMIGHTYE, eternall, impassible, and incomprehen-
sible Lorde God, whiche haste created all thinges of
nothinge, and man out of the slime of the earthe, set-

tinge him in paradyse to live ever in felicitye, from whiche he most disobedientlye fell into this worlde of infyrmities; whiche infirmities yet neverthelesse thou haste, (of thy greate mercye), so pityed, that for the helpe and curation of them, thou haste, (by thy speciall grace), geven vertue unto trees, herbes, rootes, beastes, foules, fishes, wormes, stones, and metalles; and in fyne hast left nothing among all that thou haste made wythout a propre vertue, for man his utilitye and helpe in tyme of neede, and haste also, moste graciouslye geven knowledge unto men for to use and minister thy creatures to the helpe of their griefes, graunte unto me, moste mercifull God, that (as I truely beleve, and faithfully trust, that all healthe and vertue commeth from thee), I maye so knowe and use thy creatures to the helpe of my Christen brethren and neighboures, in that arte that I, throughe thy providence, Lave from my youthe up bene trained and instituted unto, that not onlye I for the prosperous successe of mine arte, but my poore pacientes also, and all other together, maye praise and honor thy holy and blessed name, which livest and reignest one God in trinitye, and trinitye in unitye, world wythout end.   Amen.

AN OTHER.

O Lorde God, everlasting and almighty chirurgien, who only art the Lord that healest Israell, (that is thine elect), and hast created medicin out of the earth, (of no wise man to be abhorred), so that bitter water was made swete by the vertue of a tree, that men

mighte learne therby to knowe that thou haste geven
vertue to all thinges, and hast geven wisdome and
knowledge unto men from time to time, that thou
maist be honored in thy wonderous workes. For Salomon spake of all rotes and trees, even from the cedar
that groweth in Libanon, unto the hisope that spring-
eth out of the wall. Ye, he spake also of beastes, foules,
wormes, and of fishes. I reade also, O Lorde, that by
a little meale, the bitternesse of colocinthis was cured
in the potage pot of the prophets children ; and by a
plaster of figges kinge Ezechias was healed of his sicknesse sore. I also remember that by the gaule of a
fyshe, the blindnesse was taken from olde Tobies eyes.
Innumerable, O Lorde, are the testimonies of scripture,
beside dailye experience, whiche provoketh and stir-
reth me to laud and praise thy moste glorious name !
I beseche thee therfore, oh moste mercifull Lord, that
I maye so use, and all my patientes so receive, thy
creatures, that thou so graciously haste ordeined for
medicine, that health may be obteined, and thy name
for the same everlastingly honored. Graunt this, Oh
Lorde, holy and everlivyng God, for the merites of
thy dere Sonne, our only Saviour and mercye seate,
thy holy wisdome Jesus Christ, in whom is all vertue
to cure all thynges, worlde without ende. Amen.

A PRAIER TO BE USED OF THE GOOD CHIRURGIEN
BEFORE HE CONCLUDE TO TAKE IN HANDE THE
CURATION OF ANY HARDE AND DIFFICULTE THING,
AT ANY MANS IMPORTUNATE SUTE AND REQUESTE.

O ALMIGHTIE Lorde God, heavenly Father, who by

E

thy divine providence forseest and disposest all thinges
to thy glory, and the profite of thy Churche.   Thou
seest all thinges before they come to pass, and thinges
that yet are not are with thee as though they were ;
but man thou hast inclosed within metes and boundes
of knowyng thinges after they are chanced, so that we
only judge of thinges present, and as for thynges to
come, we can not before hande certenly decerne them.
Not withstanding for so much as thou hast mercifully
decreed through our Lorde Jesus Christe, that all
thinges turne to the beste to those thy chosen chyldren,
who rightly love and feare thee.   Thy strengthe sup-
plieth our weakenes, thy wysdome our folye, and thy
knowledge our ignorance ; and causest us, neverthelesse, to fele by faithe in our soules, that whiche our
carnall senses can in no wyse taste.   My prayer, therfore, oh mercifull Lorde, is that of thy gracious goodnes, and merciful benignitie, thou wilt so forsee and
provide for me, most unworthy and wretched sinner,
(yet thy servant through Christe), that I never take
upon me to cure either this, or any other thing, unles
thy godly will be, that I may through thy grace so
ende the same that not only I may thereby attayne an
honest fame, and the partie greved joye, gladnes, and
health; but chiefly that we both, and all other good
people, (the same consideryng), may remember thee
with thankes, laud, honor, and prayse, for thyne abun-
dant mercie, grace, and vertue, to our lyves ende.
Graunt this, O Lorde God, eternall and omnipotent,
for the sake of thy everlasting word, thy dere Sonne,

our only Saviour and Mediatour, by whome thou workest all in all thynges, who lyveth and reigneth with
thee and the Holy Ghost, one God in trinitie, and trinitie in unitie, worlde without end. Amen.

———

Nowe that after my symple skill I have formed
praiers mete for chirurgiens, I thinke it mete to shew
also an example howe to prayse God for the good
successe of the chirurgiens busines, as foloweth.

O ETERNALL father, almyghtie God, maker of al things,
howe great and glorious are all thy wonderous workes,
thy lovyng kyndnes and mercies to mankynde excedynge
them all, for thy benefites bestowed on mankynde are
infinite and incomparable. Among whiche thy creatures and workes of thy handes, I, moste poore unworthy man, and wretched sinner, have endlesse cause to
acknowledge thy grace and mercies.

If, oh Lord, I should once imagin to gratifie thy
goodnes, beholde what hath mortal man to geve unto
God? or what hath man that is not Gods? neyther
hast thou, O God, any nede of man, or ought that man
hath. But not withstandyng, thy Sonne our Saviour,
by divyne providence, hath satisfied for us thy wyll,
and apeased thy wrath, justly bente on us for our ma-
nifold sinnes, and through the Holy Ghoste, thy spirit
of truthe, (who leadeth us unto all truthe), we are in-
formed that thou askeste of us from henceforthe no
more, but a lyvely sacrifice of thankes gevyng and
prayse of thy holy name.

Wherfore not withstanding mine unworthines, through Christe I am boldened, (fully hopyng that of thy great mercye thou wilt fatherly accepte the same), moste hartily to thanke thee with all my harte and soule, for the good successe that haste geven to the exercise of my handes to bringe even wonderfull thinges to passe. Wherfore, O Lorde, holy and just, all possible thankes, honour, glory, and prayse, be geven unto thee. Beseching thee, (for Jesus Christes sake), to geve me grace that I never forgette or put out of mynde for any thynge whyle I lyve, to remember styll to offer thee this sacrifice, so that I receyve not this thy great graces unthankefully unto my lyves end; and after this lyfe that I may with the holy patriarkes, prophetes, apostles, evangelistes, martyrs, confessors, angels, and archangels, synge with incessant voyce before thy throne, holy, holy, holy, Lorde God of Sabaoth, for ever and ever.   Amen.

Finally, see that ye ascribe al honor unto the holy Trinitie, and seke not in any wyse your owne prayse and vayne glorie, least ye therin displease God, and justely provoke hym to withdrawe his grace frome you, whose instrumentes ye are, whyle ye dooe well, as is the hammer in the hande of the woorke manne.   For as sayeth the prophete Esaie, (cap. 10.) *Num gloriabitur securis adversus eum qui ea secat? aut serra magnificabitur adversus eum qui se tractat?   Quod perinde esset ac si virga sese elevaret contra eum qui ipsam fert, et baculus sese extolleret quasi lignum non esset.*   That

is, shall the axe boste it selfe against him that heweth therwith? or shall the sawe bragge against
him that handleth it?   Whiche were
even lyke as if the rodde did exalte
it selfe against hym that beareth it, and the staffe should
extolle it selfe as
though it weare
no woode.

FINIS.

NOTES.

P. 3, l. 1.—*Epistle and Prefaces.* These allude to the work of Lanfranc, to the translation of which, by John Halle, the " Historiall Expostulation" is appended.

P. 3, l. 16,—*Daphnoydes.* Δαφνοειδὴς, the Greek term for the laurel plant.

P. 5, l. 10.—*Blind Bayerd, or Bayard.* Bayard signifies properly a bay horse, and is sometimes used for a horse in general. " As bold as blind Bayard," is to be found in Ray's Collection of Proverbs, alluding to a person who leaps before he looks ; and Chaucer (edit. Urry, p. 126.)

> " Though ye prolle aye, ye shall it nevir find,
> Ye ben as bolde as is *bayarde the blinde*."

P. 16, l. 20.—*Eliotes bookes.* This must be an allusion to Sir Thomas Elyot, an eminent scholar in the reign of Henry VIII, who excelled in the knowledge of grammar, rhetoric, philosophy, physic, and history. He died in 1546, having, besides other works, written " The Governour," " The Castle of Helthe," " Of the Education of Children," " The Banquet of Sapience." The only medical work he published was the Castle of Health, which went through many editions, printed by Berthelet, Marshe, and others, and which subjected him to much censure from members of the medical profession, as well

as the community in general. The latter conceived it to
be a subject beneath the dignity of the pen of a knight,
and the former were incensed that it should be written in
English. Sir Thomas Elyot was one of the most learned
and virtuous men of his time, and an intimate of Sir
Thomas More.

P. 18, l. 3.—*Maister Luke, of London, hath a great name for
curyng eyes.* I can find no other notice of this practi-
tioner; he does not appear to have published any work,
or detailed his modes of practice. Several interesting
notices of quack oculists will be found in Mr. Rim-
bault's edition of Chettle's " Kind-Hearts Dreame,"
printed by the Percy Society (pp. 22-26-75.) I have also
given several in a Memoir of the late James Ware, Esq.
See Medical Portrait Gallery, vol. iii.

P. 19, l. 27.—*Maister Vicary.* Thomas Vicary was one of
the earliest writers on anatomy in the English language.
He was serjeant-surgeon to four sovereigns, namely:
Henry VIII, Edward VI, and queens Mary and Elizabeth. He was also chief surgeon to St. Bartholomew's
Hospital, the principal scene of his labours. In 1548 he
published " The Englishman's Treasure, with the true
Anatomy of Man's Body," London, 4to. This was several times reprinted, and an edition with the title somewhat altered, was put forth in 1577, by the surgeons of
St. Bartholomew's Hospital.

P. 21, l. 13.—*He answered Vigo, and Gasken.* Of the latter
nothing is known. John de Vigo was physician to Pope
Julius II, and wrote largely and wisely on several sub-
jects of surgery. He composed many treatises, the whole
of which were collected together, and translated into

56

NOTES.

English by Bartholomew Traheron, and published in
folio, in 1543, and again in 1550, from the press of
Edward Whytchurch ; it was reprinted in 1571, by
Thomas East, and Henry Middelton, and again in 1586,
4to., together with some pieces by Thomas Gale, with a
preface by George Baker, Gent., who together with
Richard Norton, diligently revised and corrected the
whole work, which was printed by Thomas East.

P. 26, l. 3.—*Grigge the Poulter.* In the reign of Edward VI,
Grigg, a poulterer in Surrey, was put in the pillory at
Croydon and again in Southwark, for cheating people
out of their money by pretending to cure them by charms,
or by looking at them, or by casting their water. (Gentle-
man's Magazine, Vol. xxxiii. p. 105). Many other
quacks have at various times been also subjected to punish-
ment.—Anthony was punished for his Aurum Potabile ;
Arthur Dee for advertising medicines to cure all diseases ;
Foster for selling a powder for the cure of chlorosis ;
Tenant, an urine caster, who sold pills at £6 each ; Aires
for selling purging sugar plums ; Hunt for putting up bills
for the cure of diseases in the streets. The Council in the
reign of James I despatched a warrant to the Magistrates
of the City of London, to take up all reputed empirics,
and cause them to be examined by the censors of the
Royal College of Physicians. Several were taken up and
acknowledged their ignorance ; Lamb, Reed, Wood-
house, &c. In the reign of King William, Fairfax was
fined and imprisoned for doing injury to persons by his
Aqua Cœlestis. And in Stow's Chronicle it is recorded
that a water caster was punished for exercising his quack-
ery. He was set on horseback, his face to the horse's tail,
which he held in his hand, with a collar of urinals about
his neck, led by the hangman through the city, whipped,
branded, and then banished.

P. 26, l. 28.—*Maister Bulleyne.* William Bulleyn, or Bullein, was a learned physician, born about the year 1500, in the Isle of Ely. He was intimately versed in the writings of the Greek and Arabian physicians, and he travelled over various parts of England and Scotland, to acquire botanical knowledge. He studied both at Cambridge and at Oxford, and was an ecclesiastic as well as a physician. He was rector of Blaxhall, in Suffolk, where he preached divinity, and practised physic. Upon the accession of Queen Mary, being a protestant, he thought it best to retire from his rectory, and he removed to Durham; where he became intimate with Sir Thomas Hilton, governor of Tinmouth Fort, engaged with him in a commercial speculation, and had occasion, also, to attend upon him in an attack of malignant fever, of which he died. Bulleyn was pursued and charged, by the brother of the governor, with the murder of his relative, but of this he was honourably acquitted. He was, however, detained in prison for a debt, and during his incarceration composed his medical works, which are distinguished by learning, fancy, and humour. They consist of "The Governement of Helthe," "A Comfortable Regimen against the Pleurisie ;" Bulwarke of Defense against all Sicknes, Sornes, and Wounds, that doe daily assaulte Mankind ;" and "A Dialogue both pleasaunt and pietieful against the Fever Pestilence." He was elected into the Royal College of Physicians of London, and had a great practice. He died in 1576.

P. 27, l. 13.—*For where as before thyne errors were espied.* This of Socrates appears to be the original of that which has been reported of others. The eccentric Dr. Radcliffe is known never to have paid his bills without much importunity ; a paviour, after long and fruitless attempts,

caught the Doctor just as he was alighting from his cha-
riot, at his own door in Bloomsbury Square, and accosted
him. " Why you rascal," said the Doctor, " do you pre-
tend to be paid for such a piece of work? why you have
spoiled my pavement, and then covered it over with
earth to hide your bad work." " Doctor," said the paviour, " mine is not the only bad work that the earth
hides." " You dog, you," said the Doctor, " are you a
wit? you must be poor, come in."—and paid him.—*See
Medical Portrait Gallery*, vol. i.

P. 38, l. 1.—*But also in Astronomye.* Sir George Ripley, in
his ' Compound of Alchimie,' tells us that—

> " A good phisytian who so intendeth to be,
>   Our lower astronomy him nedeth well to knowe ;
> And after that to lerne, well, urine in a a glasse to see,
>   And if it neede to be chafed the fyre to blowe,
> Then wyttily it, by divers wayes to throwe,
>   And after the cause to make a medicine blive,
> Truly telling the ynfirmities all on a rowe :
>   Who thus can doe by his physicke is like to thrive."

Chaucer's picture of a good physician, will furnish also
another instance of the prevalent opinion of the necessity
of a knowledge of astronomy, in practitioners of the
medical art. I have adduced many other authorities in
my work " On Superstitions connected with the History
and Practice of Medicine and Surgery."

P. 41, l. 14.—*Angelus Bolognius.* Angelo Bolognini was an
Italian surgeon and professor of surgery at Padua, from
1508 to 1517. He is generally regarded as the inventor
of the use of mercurial frictions. The able work of this
surgeon referred to by Halle, is inserted in the collection
of Gesner and Uffenbach, entitled " De cura Ulcerum
exteriorum et de Unguentis communibus in Solutione
continui."

P. 42, l. 17.—*Good Doctor Record.* Robert Recorde, doctor
of medicine, is a person of whom we have to regret that
but few biographical particulars are known. My friend
Mr. James Orchard Halliwell has, in an interesting
little tract on "The connexion of Wales with the early
science of England," published by Rodd in 1840, collected together several circumstances which show that he
is to be regarded as the first original writer on arithmetic
in English; the first on geometry; the first person who
introduced the knowledge of algebra into England; the
first writer on astronomy in English; the first person in
this country who adopted the Copernican system; the
inventor of the present method of extracting the square
root; the inventor of the sign of equality; and the inventor of the method of extracting the square root of
multinomial algebraic quantities. He lived in the reigns
of Henry VIII, Edward VI, and Queen Mary; to the
latter sovereign he was physician. He was a native of
Tenby in Pembrokeshire, and, according to Fuller, a
protestant: he publicly taught rhetoric, mathematics,
music, and anatomy, at Oxford, about the year 1525, and
was elected a fellow of All Souls College in 1531. He was
created M.D. at Cambridge in 1545, resided in London
in 1547, and is supposed to have died in 1558. His will,
from which Mr. Halliwell has given some extracts, bears
the date of June 28, 1558, and he therein styles himself
as "sicke in body, yet whole in mynde." This will
was made in the King's Bench prison, where he was
confined a prisoner for debt. His works, which are
all written in the form of Dialogue between pupil and
teacher, consist of "The Grounde of Artes;" (arithmetic);
"The Urinall of Physick;" (a work entitled "the Judicial
of Urines" is supposed to be the same with a different
title; I have never been able to see a copy of it). "The

Pathway to Knowledge," (Geometry); " The Gate of Knowledge," (Mensuration); " The Castel of Knowledge," (Astrology and Mathematics); " The Treasure of Knowledge," (Astronomy); " The Whetstone of Witte," (Algebra and Arithmetic). All these were printed between the years 1540, and 1557, and most of them several times reprinted. Recorde also edited the early edition of Fabyan's Chronicle, and Sherburne attributes to him " Cosmographiæ Isagoge," " De Arte Faciendi Horologium," and " De Usu Globorum et de Statu Temporum." He is said to have been well skilled in the Saxon language, and to have made large collections of historical and other ancient manuscripts.

P. 42, l. 25.—*As Guido saythe.* Guy de Chauliac was in surgical science one of the most distinguished men of the 14th century. He studied at Bologna, and at Montpellier, where he afterwards was appointed a professor. He practised at Lyons, and was physician to Pope Clement VI in 1348. He has given an excellent account of the plague as it appeared at Avignon. His principal efforts were directed to the improvement of surgery, which he relieved from many of the barbarous practices of his age. He improved the method of performing many operations, and invented several instruments. His works were collected together, and published as Chirurgiæ Tractatus Septem cum Antidotario, which first appeared at Venice in 1490, and was afterwards published under the editorial care of several surgeons, and repeatedly printed.

RICHARDS, PRINTER, ST. MARTIN'S LANE.

Printed in the United States
By Bookmasters